D1261774

Weight Watchers®
Tools for Living Journal

MACMILLAN
A Simon & Schuster Macmillan Company
1633 Broadway
New York, NY 10019

Copyright © 1998 Weight Watchers International, Inc.

All rights reserved. No part of this book may be reproduced or transmitted in any form by any means, electronic or mechanical, including photocopying, recording, or by any information storage and retrieval system, without permission of the publisher.

A Word About Weight Watchers

Since 1963, Weight Watchers has grown from a handful of people to millions of enrollees annually. Today, Weight Watchers is recognized as the leading name in safe and sensible weight control. Weight Watchers members form a diverse group, from youths to senior citizens, attending meetings virtually around the globe.

Weight-loss and weight-management results vary by individual, but we recommend that you attend Weight Watchers meetings, follow the Weight Watchers food plan and participate in regular physical activity. For the Weight Watchers meeting nearest you, call 1-800-651-6000.

Weight Watchers Publishing Group

Editorial Director: Nancy Gagliardi

Senior Editor: Martha Schueneman

Associate Editor: Christine Senft, M.S.

Text: Barbara Turvett

MACMILLAN is a registered trademark of Macmillan, Inc.

WEIGHT WATCHERS is a registered trademark of Weight Watchers International, Inc.

Library of Congress Cataloging-in-Publication Data available

ISBN 0-02-862877-2

Manufactured in the United States of America

10 9 8 7 6 5 4 3 2 1

Design by Christine Weathersbee

Welcome to Your Journal

You are about to do a wonderful thing for yourself. It is something that can help you relax, understand yourself, get organized and achieve your goals. It is something that is fun. It is something that offers you a safe and private haven for heart and soul. And it is something that can help you manage your issues with food and weight. You are about to begin a journal.

Quite simply, a journal is a place to write down your innermost thoughts and feelings. You can also record your impressions of things happening in and around your life and write down any new ideas or revelations occurring to you. You can express yourself with long passages, or you can write just isolated words or brief statements. You can sketch in your journal, write a poem, record something you've heard or read, or write whatever words come into your mind during a moment of free association. You can carry it with you, perhaps to Weight Watchers meetings, and use it to take notes or jot down relevant ideas that you've heard. The point is that there are no rules to writing in a journal. It is your private place in which to do what you want. It is not "one more thing you have to do," but rather a place where you can be relaxed and free.

What is the Weight Watchers Tools for Living Journal?

Why is this journal different? Because it focuses on strategies to help you achieve your goals—Weight Watchers Tools for Living. These Tools, and this journal, can help you manage your thoughts and feelings about your weight-loss efforts. The Tools are:

Winning Outcomes: A Winning Outcome is a specific goal that is stated in the positive, fits your lifestyle, and that you can do on your own. An example of a short-term Winning Outcome is: "I want to keep my eating under control at the party this weekend." A long-term Winning Outcome is: "I want to follow the Weight Watchers program so I can achieve lasting weight loss and feel healthy and good about myself."

Empowering Beliefs: These are ideas that you believe are true, the ones coming from deep within you, helping you achieve your goals. For example, "I will lose weight and feel better about myself because I am worth it," is an Empowering Belief.

Anchoring: This is a technique that helps you call up your personal strengths and characteristics whenever you need them to achieve something. By remembering a past event that made you feel powerful, and then deciding upon an object, word or image to remind you of the event and the feeling of power, you can focus on the object at any time to recall that positive feeling.

Storyboarding: A Storyboard is a step-by-step action plan that you draw up, much like a sequence of scenes in a film, to help you get closer to a goal. An example of the steps leading to the goal "I want to lose weight and feel more energetic" could be: (1) Join Weight Watchers; (2) Follow the Food Plan; (3) Track what I eat; (4) Go to meetings weekly; (5) Exercise for 20 minutes every day.

Mental Rehearsing: This is a practice in which you create an imaginary movie in your mind that has you doing what you want to do in a given situation. Say, for instance, you are going to your parents' for the weekend, but you don't want to fall into old, detrimental eating habits while there. You imagine yourself eating moderately at each meal, as you happily say "No thanks, Mom" to extra helpings and rich, heavy foods. You see yourself having a calm conversation with your mother about the new eating habits you're developing.

Motivating Strategy: This is another mental practice to inspire your continued efforts toward a Winning Outcome. Imagine that you've already achieved a goal, such as losing 30 pounds. Visualize yourself at the office, giving a presentation, dressed in a fabulous designer suit, feeling confident about the way you look and feel, receiving high praise from your colleagues for your presentation. Take a moment to bask in the good feelings you are experiencing, and then remember the feelings as you continue to move toward your goal.

Reframing: With this Tool, you can find positive behaviors to take the place of negative ones. If, for example, you eat when you feel bored at night, write down several other things you can do to eliminate evening ennui, such as reading an exciting novel, calling an old friend and gabbing, going to the gym or surfing the Web. Then choose three ideas you like and try one tonight. If that one doesn't work, try another. Remember, you always have a choice to do something other than eating.

Positive Self-Talking: Thinking, speaking and writing positive thoughts to yourself is a sure road to positive action. To help you achieve your goals, you can: List your life successes, congratulate yourself on your daily accomplishments and replace negative thoughts with positive ones (instead of "My weight loss is going so slowly," write "My jeans are getting baggier.").

Scattered throughout the pages of this journal are symbols that represent the Tools for Living. These symbols, plus the tips you'll also find sprinkled about, are there to stimulate your journal-writing success. Use them to help you address issues that crop up day to day. Allow them to keep you focused on your journey to healthy eating and a healthy life.

Why Keep a Journal?

Writing in your journal will take some time out of your busy day, but there are many valuable benefits to be gained from keeping a journal.

Self-expression and understanding: Writing down your feelings—about people, work, food, your body, anything, in fact—allows you to look more objectively at what is going on in your head and your heart. When your thoughts are down on paper, you can reflect upon and evaluate them in terms of how things in your life affect you. Examining your feelings also can help you clarify your wants and needs. Then you can decide if you need to make changes. In this way, your journal becomes a tool for self-exploration, one that many have found to be highly effective.

Motivation: Your journal is an excellent place to list goals, both short- and long-term. Making lists of things you want to accomplish, and then checking off the items you've achieved, can help you to get things done. Seeing a list of wants and needs also can help you prioritize them.

Problem-solving: Writing in your journal will allow you to examine obstacles and look for ways to overcome them. Sometimes you may not be able to pinpoint a problem in your mind, but by writing out your feelings when you feel upset, the true problem will reveal itself. Once you see the issue in words, you're more able to address it. You can examine its causes and effects. Then you can list any and all possible solutions to the problem and ask yourself what the positive and negative consequences of each solution are. By listing various solutions to a problem, and their pros and cons, you can arrive at the one that works best for you.

Stress relief: Studies have shown that writing helps relieve tension and stress. It's not surprising, then, that venting frustration is one of the most common reasons people write in journals. Expressing strong emotions on paper can help release some of the pent-up feelings within you. It is also a way to examine the feelings that create stress and to look for their causes and resolutions.

Organization: Keeping a food log in your journal can keep you organized about what foods, situations and feelings trigger your overeating, and help you determine the way you want to eat, day by day.

Creative expression: By allowing yourself, freely and regularly, to express your individuality through writing and drawing in your journal, you open up your creative self. You can explore your dreams and desires. You can record the wonderful things you experience each day. You can give rise, without judging yourself, to any creative impulses. In this way, you enhance your relationship with your inner self. And the stronger this relationship is, the more you will love yourself, feel worthy and decrease the need to comfort yourself with food.

How to Use this Journal

Remember that there are no hard-and-fast rules to keeping a journal. Let yourself be guided by the things you want to accomplish. Allow yourself to work things out on paper when they are nagging you. Don't worry if answers are slow to reveal themselves to you. As you release your feelings on paper, you'll get the immediate benefit of stress reduction. And more than likely, clarity about particular issues will come.

Perhaps the most difficult thing about journal writing is getting started. So put all those excuses—"I don't have time; I'm not a good writer; It seems silly to me"—behind you and just do it.

Let your creative juices flow without censorship. Scribble, doodle, vent, discuss, describe. Ask yourself questions, even if you don't answer them. There are no rules about when, or how often, you should write. Find out what works best for you. Once you're into it, you won't remember why you ever resisted it.

Celebrate Your Successes

Clearly, journal writing has benefits for everybody. But as a tool for helping bring about lasting change in your weight and the way you relate to food—and, indeed, lasting change in your life—keeping a journal has particular pluses. One important way your journal can promote your quest is by functioning as a victory log. In it, you can chronicle your achievements, successes, positive thoughts about yourself—any feelings and ideas that serve to applaud your efforts. There are many easy and fun ways to do this; here are a few suggestions:

Describe a happy occasion. Write about a goal you've accomplished, or something wonderful that has happened, or even a small victory you experienced that day. Be as brief or as detailed as you like. You'll feel as happy while you write about it as when you experienced it—and you can feel the joy each time you reread the entry.

Make a list. Each day, week or every few days, make a list of each good thing you've experienced during that time period. This can include those times you ate healthfully, lost weight, helped somebody, stuck to your food plan, played with your children, had a good day at work—whatever.

Write down your fine points. Jot down one, two or three things you like about yourself—your kindness, your haircut, your eyes, your weight loss over the last month. Draw boxes around these for extra focus.

Just picture it. Every time you feel particularly good about the way you eat, draw one little picture that is your key to that good feeling. It could be a flower, a happy face, a star . . . you get the idea. When you flip through the pages of your journal and see this charming visual, you'll be reminded of how often you've succeeded.

Remember that there is no right or wrong way to keep a journal. Whether you're apt to write just a few sketchy words or lengthy paragraphs of prose, the idea is to be honest and true to yourself. You'll benefit from whatever way you choose to recognize your strengths and accomplishments.

Explore the Tough Stuff

Writing in your journal can help you look at the issues in your life that confuse you or cause you pain—issues that are perhaps leading you to overeat. Through your writing, you can confront these issues, dissect and examine them, and also explore possible resolutions. You can see obstacles to your weight loss as they arise. Working out these troubles in your journal will allow you to separate them from yourself. In other words, you'll be able to see them as your behaviors, not as who you are. You can analyze the problems objectively, without blaming or beating up yourself.

In addition to writing, drawing pictures that reflect your fears, problems, obstacles and feelings can be helpful. Do whatever feels comfortable.

Back to the Future

Life is a process, a journey. By writing in a journal, you give yourself a record of that journey. It is an intimate, detailed chronicle of your personal growth. When you write about something, it is yours to keep, to remember. Granted, a lot of what you put in your journal will be plain, everyday thoughts. Some of the passages will be about painful things: hard times, tough emotions, negative thoughts about yourself and others. But intertwined will be joyous things: hurdles overcame, battles won, milestones reached, happy times, exciting insights.

Each time you go back to read through your journal, you'll remind yourself that yours is a life of ups and downs, successes and slips, highs and lows. But one thing will be clear: You are growing as a human being. Your journal will show your progress in all areas of your life. And reviewing your past growth will serve only to encourage your continued growth and enhance your weight-loss success!

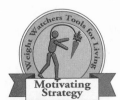

Write down the "dream"
you want to realize.

Weight Watchers Tools for Living

Motivating
Strategy

_____

_____

_____

_____

_____

_____

_____

_____

_____

_____

_____

_____

_____

I am a slow walker, but I never walk back.
Abraham Lincoln

Tip: Describe a beautiful
thing you saw today.

_____

_____

_____

_____

_____

_____

_____

_____

_____

_____

_____

_____

_____

_____

_____

_____

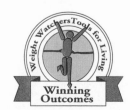

Write down your long-term
Winning Outcome.

Tip: Before you write, take a few deep breaths
to clear your mind and center yourself.

Whether you think you can, or whether
you think you can't, you're right!
Henry Ford

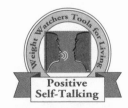

Positive self-talk for today:
"I can, I can, I can!"

Positive
Self-Talking

Tip: Today, use pictures instead of words
to express all your thoughts and feelings.

_____

_____

_____

_____

_____

_____

_____

_____

_____

_____

_____

_____

_____

_____

Choice, not chance, determines destiny.

Anonymous

_____

_____

_____

_____

_____

_____

_____

_____

_____

_____

_____

_____

_____

_____

_____

_____

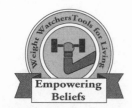

You are a unique human being and
you deserve to achieve your goals.

Tip: Try writing outdoors today,
allowing nature's beauty to inspire you.

_____

_____

_____

_____

_____

_____

_____

_____

_____

_____

_____

_____

_____

Tip: Describe how you would like
to feel about food and eating.

_____

_____

_____

_____

_____

_____

_____

_____

_____

_____

_____

_____

_____

_____

_____

_____

_____

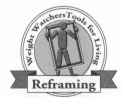

Think of three things to do instead of snacking on food when you're upset.

_____

_____

_____

_____

_____

_____

_____

_____

_____

_____

_____

_____

_____

_____

_____

You have to let go of what you thought you
were to discover what you really are.
Anonymous

_____

_____

_____

_____

_____

_____

_____

_____

_____

_____

_____

_____

_____

_____

_____

_____

_____

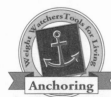 To help you meet a challenge, remind yourself of your inner strengths.

_____

_____

_____

_____

_____

_____

_____

_____

_____

_____

_____

_____

_____

_____

_____

_____

_____

_____

_____

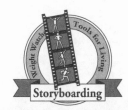

Set a Winning Outcome for the
end of the week, and write a
Storyboard to help you achieve it.

Tip: Start your writing today with this sentence:
"Today is a new beginning."

_____

_____

_____

_____

_____

_____

_____

_____

_____

_____

_____

_____

_____

_____

Tip: Write a short letter to someone and
discuss how you want to feel about yourself.

_____

_____

_____

_____

_____

_____

_____

_____

_____

_____

_____

_____

_____

_____

_____

_____

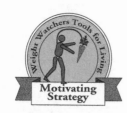

Imagine yourself feeling great
as you finish a three-mile walk.
Write how you feel.

_____

_____

_____

_____

_____

_____

_____

_____

_____

_____

_____

_____

_____

We cannot direct the wind, but we can adjust our sails.

Anonymous

_____

_____

_____

_____

_____

_____

_____

_____

_____

_____

_____

_____

Tip: Think about a recent overeating episode;
write down your feelings about it.

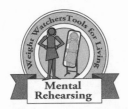

Write out a mini-screenplay so you can mentally rehearse an important upcoming event.

You can't solve a problem in
the mind-set that created it.
Albert Einstein

No man is an island entire unto himself.

John Donne

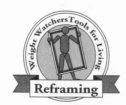

There is always another choice.

_____

_____

_____

_____

_____

_____

_____

_____

_____

_____

_____

_____

_____

_____

Tip: Draw a picture of how you want to look.

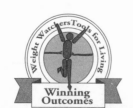

Focus on what you want.

_____

_____

_____

_____

_____

_____

_____

_____

_____

_____

_____

_____

_____

_____

_____

Tip: Write down any questions that come into
your mind. Then see where they take you.

People are generally better persuaded by
the reasons which they themselves discovered,
than by those which come into the minds of others.
Pascal

_____

_____

_____

_____

_____

_____

_____

_____

_____

_____

_____

_____

_____

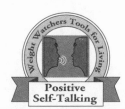

Write down a weight-loss
victory of the day.

We are what we repeatedly do.

Excellence, then, is not an act, but a habit.

Aristotle

_____

_____

_____

_____

_____

_____

_____

_____

_____

_____

_____

_____

_____

Tip: List those feelings that are
hard for you to express.

_____

_____

_____

_____

_____

_____

_____

_____

_____

_____

_____

_____

_____

_____

_____

_____

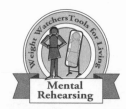

Write out how you'd like
to look, feel and act
at an upcoming event.

_____

_____

_____

_____

_____

_____

_____

_____

_____

_____

_____

Living the past is dull and lonely business;
looking back strains the neck muscles, causes
you to bump into people not going your way.
Edna Ferber

_____

_____

_____

_____

_____

_____

_____

_____

_____

_____

_____

_____

_____

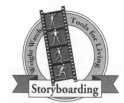

Describe the path to your dream.

It's easier to say what we believe
than to be what we believe.
Anonymous

Tip: If you write it down, it's yours to keep.

_____

_____

_____

_____

_____

_____

_____

_____

_____

_____

_____

_____

_____

_____

_____

_____

_____

_____

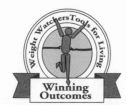 Being clear about what you want
helps you achieve it.

Tip: Make a list of all the feelings
you have about food.

Tip: Have a dialogue with your body.

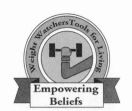
Empowering
Beliefs

Start your journal today with
this sentence: "I'm worth it!"

No one can make us feel inferior

without our consent.

Eleanor Roosevelt

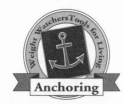

Describe a time you felt strong and in control; then create a reminder of that feeling for the future.

_____

_____

_____

_____

_____

_____

_____

_____

_____

_____

_____

_____

_____

_____

_____

If you find a path with no obstacles,
it probably doesn't lead anywhere.

Anonymous

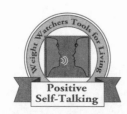

**Positive
Self-Talking**

We are what we eat.

We are what we repeat.

There is nothing either good or bad,

but thinking makes it so.

William Shakespeare

_____

_____

_____

_____

_____

_____

_____

_____

_____

_____

_____

_____

_____

_____

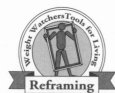 Fill in the blank: "Instead of eating to calm myself, I will _____ today."

Tip: Write down ten things
you're grateful for.

. . . As long as one keeps searching, the answers come.

Joan Baez

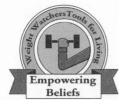

Empowering Beliefs

You have the power to make lasting changes in your life.

The self is not something ready-made, but something
in continuous formation through choice of action.
John Dewey

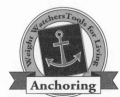

Anchoring

You have all the resources you
need to reach your goals.

Human beings, by changing the inner attitudes of their
minds, can change the outer aspects of their lives.
William James

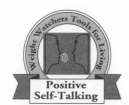

Weight Watchers Tools for Living

Positive
Self-Talking

List three things you
like about yourself.

_____

_____

_____

_____

_____

_____

_____

_____

_____

_____

_____

_____

_____

_____

Tip: Feel pride in how far you've come and
confidence in where you are going.

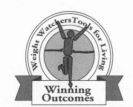

Winning Outcomes

What do you want?

_____

_____

_____

_____

_____

_____

_____

_____

_____

_____

_____

_____

_____

Nothing in life is to be feared.

It is only to be understood.

Marie Curie

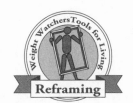

There's no such thing as
failure, only feedback.

Accept the challenges so that you
may feel the exhilaration of victory.
General George S. Patton

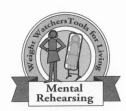

Mentally rehearse eating out at
a fine restaurant, and write
how you feel afterward.

Tip: Go back and read all of
your journal entries to date.

If you don't scale the mountain, you can't see the view.

Anonymous

_____

_____

_____

_____

_____

_____

_____

_____

_____

_____

_____

_____

_____

_____

_____

_____

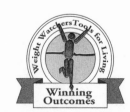

Revisit and revise your
Winning Outcomes.

_____

_____

_____

_____

_____

_____

_____

_____

_____

_____

_____

_____

_____

Tip: If you can imagine it, you can achieve it.
If you can dream it, you can become it.

Journal writing is a voyage to the interior.
Christina Baldwin

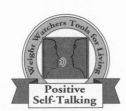

Positive Self-Talking

List 100 things that
are good in your life.

All the flowers of all the tomorrows
are in the seeds of today.
Anonymous

With time and patience, the mulberry
leaf becomes a silk gown.
Chinese proverb

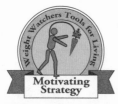

We move toward what we
picture in our minds.